anita bean's

six week workout

LOVELY LEGS

D1079477

Before starting this or any other exercise programme, you should check with your doctor if you have any health problems, are taking medication, are recovering from an injury or illness or if you haven't taken exercise for over a year.

While the advice and information in this book is believed to be accurate and up to date, it is advisory only and should not be used as an alternative to seeking specialist medical advice. The author and publishers cannot be held responsible for any injury sustained while following the exercises or using the information contained in this book, which are taken entirely at the reader's own risk.

Published in 2005 by A & C Black Publishers Ltd
37 Soho Square, London W1D 3QZ
www.acblack.com

Copyright © 2005 by Anita Bean

ISBN 0 7136 7199 8

Acknowledgements
Cover photography
Illustrations by James
Text photography by

Printed and bound in

contents

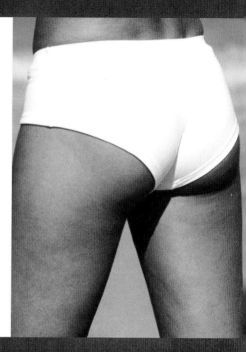

acknowledgements

Many thanks to my husband Simon, and daughters Chloe and Lucy, for all their support. A big thank you to photographer Grant Pritchard, personal trainer Steve Tunstall (www.stpersonaltraining.co.uk) for demonstrating the exercises, and my editors at A & C Black, Claire Dunn and Hannah McEwen.

Photos were shot on location at Holmes Place, Epsom.

introduction

Much like a love of shopping or chocolate cravings, a desire for sexier, leaner legs is something we all share. And the great news is that, no matter how long or short your legs, you can dramatically improve their shape. The secret lies in a smart combination of exercise and diet.

It seems unfair that, for most women, any surplus body fat goes straight on the hips and thighs, hence the classic pear shape. Even when you manage to lose weight from elsewhere, the hips and thighs often stay flabby. Worse, this spare flab often appears as that dimply, wobbly, 'orange peel' fat we call cellulite. According to one survey, 95 per cent of women over 30 say they have cellulite. It seems to affect thin women and fit women. Even A-list celebs get it

The key to flab-free, toned thighs is a three-pronged attack:

◼ cardiovascular (CV) exercise to burn fat (including cellulite) and stimulate the circulation

◼ effective toning moves like squats and lunges to up your quota of firm muscle tissue

◼ a healthy diet plan to keep your whole body in great condition.

During the next six weeks, you will be doing a combination of CV (fat-burning) and toning workouts that target your legs. Some of the exercises utilise gym machines but many can be performed at home with no or only minimal equipment, such as an exercise ball or a pair of light dumbbells. You'll also be devoting time at the end of each workout to some great stretching moves – this will help lengthen the muscles and maintain your flexibility.

This is a progressive programme designed to get you fit and keep you fit. Each week you'll be learning new exercises and doing new workouts. This will keep your muscles constantly challenged and help you stay motivated. Stick with this programme, and in six weeks you'll have your loveliest legs ever.

1 countdown

Before you start this six-week programme, you need to learn when is the best time to exercise, how to perform each move and how often you need to work out for the best results. This chapter gives you crucial tips and provides answers to the most commonly asked questions about exercising legs.

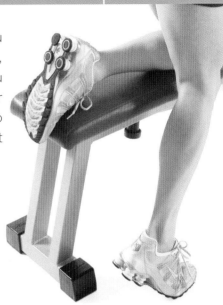

your legs

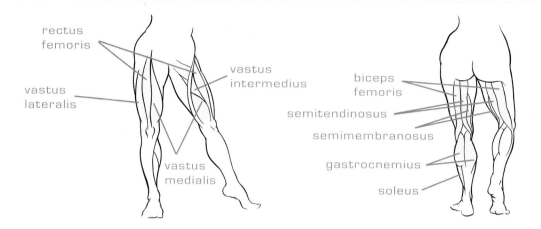

rectus
femoris

vastus
lateralis

vastus
intermedius

vastus
medialis

biceps
femoris

semitendinosus

semimembranosus

gastrocnemius

soleus

the leg muscles

The muscle at the front of the thigh, known as the **quadriceps**, consists of four parts:

1 The **rectus femoris** can be seen when the leg is lifted up and forward slightly.
2 The **vastus lateralis** runs down the outside of the thigh and can be seen on the outside of the knee.
3 The **vastus medialis** runs along the inside of the thigh to the rectus femoris and can be seen on the inside of the knee when the leg is locked out.
4 The **vastus intermedius** cannot be readily seen as it lies underneath the other muscles.

The collective function of these muscles is to extend (straighten) the knee. The rectus femoris also flexes the hip (lifts the thigh up and forwards).

The main inner-thigh muscles are comprised of three **adductor muscles** – adductor brevis, adductor longus and adductor magnus – whose function is to adduct or pull the legs together, while the muscles of the outer thigh – the gluteus minimus and gluteus medius – pull the legs out sideways.

The muscles at the back of the leg – **the hamstrings** – include the biceps femoris (long and short heads), semitendinosus and semimembranosus. They have two main actions: to flex (bend) the knee and extend the hip (pull the thigh backwards).

The **calves** are comprised of two muscles: the **gastrocnemius** and **soleus**. The gastrocnemius is the larger of the two and lies on top of the soleus. It is worked when the leg is fully straight, and has two distinct lobes, which are visible from behind when the calf is flexed. Its role is to straighten the ankle (plantar flexion), to point the toes, and it also helps bend the knee. The soleus is a broad, flat muscle, which also helps straighten the ankle. It sweeps out to the sides and over the shins, and is worked when the knee is bent at about 90 degrees.

exercise tips

work out on an empty stomach

CV exercise performed first thing in the morning on an empty stomach burns more fat than at any other time. That's because insulin levels are at their lowest and glucagon levels are at their highest. This encourages your body to draw on its fat reserves for fuel. If you work out after eating your body will use this food for fuel instead. Exercising first thing in the morning also helps kick-start your metabolism so you'll burn more calories during the rest of the day.

do cv exercise and weights on separate days

If you want to build muscle mass as well as burn fat, try to do your CV workout on a different day from weights. Research suggests that overall calorie expenditure is greater if CV and weight-training exercise are done on separate days. That's because each time you train, your metabolism is boosted – so training on most days of the week will lead to faster fat loss. But if you have to do both in one session, complete your weight-training workout first when glycogen stores are high. Do it the other way round and you risk lower strength and muscle mass gains.

keep it slow

Do each toning movement in a slow and controlled manner. This increases the intensity of the contraction and minimises injury risk. It's better to perform slower, intense movements with good control, holding each contraction for a count of two, than rushing to perform more repetitions. Use the recommended rep ranges in the workouts as a guide. If you can do more, try slowing the movement or using extra weights to make the exercise harder. When it starts to hurt (not to be confused with actual pain), move on to the next exercise.

keep your tummy in!

Keep your tummy muscles (abdominals) taut all the time. Think about gently drawing your navel towards your spine and keeping the lower portion of your tummy as flat as you can – without creating excessive tension or holding your breath. Maintain a neutral alignment of the spine at all times – think about keeping the natural 'S' contour.

good posture

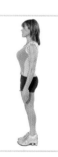

To find your neutral posture, where your joints are aligned correctly to each other, stand with your feet hip-width apart, knees relaxed. Let your shoulders drop down and away from your ears. Lengthen your spine and neck – imagine a string, attached to the top of your head, pulling you up to the ceiling. Contract your abdominal muscles, drawing your navel in towards your spine. Adjust the tilt of your pelvis so that it is in a neutral position.

go all the way

Aim to perform each toning exercise with a full range of movement, really squeezing the muscles.

breathe right

Breathe in during the easier part of the movement and breathe out during the contraction (hard part of the movement).

work legs two or three times a week

Training your legs two or three times a week is sufficient. Working them more frequently won't necessarily produce better results, and risks over-training and injury. If your legs are still sore, it's too soon to train them again.

variety is key

You should always include a variety of exercises in your leg routine to target each group of muscles and prevent them from becoming too used to the same exercises. The six workouts in this book will make sure you work each part of your legs effectively.

Q & A - *frequently asked questions*

Despite doing a lot of walking, I still have cellulite. Is it different from ordinary fat and how can I get rid of it?

You might be reassured to learn that cellulite affects 85 per cent of women, and over 95 per cent of women over 30. But cellulite is just fat. Specifically, it's fat that's stored just beneath your skin. The reason it appears dimpled and puckered is that it is criss-crossed by weak collagen strands that don't do a very good job supporting the fat cells. This results in the characteristic bulging appearance of cellulite on your body. It affects women far more than men partly because women have higher levels of oestrogen, which favours fat storage on the thighs and bottom, and partly because women have weaker connective fibres.

Inactivity and excess calories also play a big role in the formation of cellulite. Walking burns calories but unless you watch what you eat you can still gain fat. More intense CV exercise will increase your calorie burn, and stimulate your blood flow and lymphatic circulation. And including toning (resistance) exercises will help maintain or build muscle, which boosts the skin's collagen fibres and prevents the puckering that causes cellulite. Together with a healthy diet and careful calorie intake, you should be able to shift that cellulite.

Help – I'm a typical pear shape! I've got a slim top half but store too much fat around my hips and thighs. How can I get rid of the fat in these areas?

Women tend to store fat more readily around the hips and thighs due to higher levels of the female hormone oestrogen. Unfortunately, it's not possible to spot-reduce fat from any area of the body but you can certainly reduce your body fat percentage by combining a more active lifestyle with a healthier calorie intake. Burning an extra 300 calories (equivalent to 30 minutes' cycling) and cutting out 200 calories (equivalent to a couple of chocolate biscuits) a day will result in fat loss of ½ kg (1 lb) a week or 2 kg (4 lb) a month. Following the toning exercises in this six-week programme will firm your leg muscles, making your hips and thighs smaller.

I'm worried that I'll get big thighs if I do any exercises with weights.

Fear not! The conditioning exercises in this six-week programme tone rather than build muscle. You'll notice your muscles get firmer, not bigger. Even adding light or moderate weights wouldn't develop muscle size. The only way you could bulk up would be using very heavy weights over a much longer period of time.

How can I reduce the size of my calves?

In women, well-muscled calves look sexy so don't beat yourself up! The only way to reduce the size of any muscle is to work it less. So, omit direct calf exercises like calf raises from your workout.

I've got fairly slim legs but they are a bit wobbly when I walk. How can I firm them up?

You can go from wobbly to firm by doing effective toning exercises that target the major muscle groups in the legs. The workouts in this six-week programme include exercises that take the muscles through a full range of motion, and research proves that this is the most efficient way of toning up. Avoid exercises that use only short-range or limited degrees of movement. If you stick to this programme, you'll get firmer legs in no time!

I'm a runner but unhappy with my straight up and down legs – how can I get them into better shape?

This is a common problem among distance runners, due mainly to a lack of muscle development (excessive running burns muscle as well as fat). You need to include toning exercises, such as squats and lunges, which work the largest muscle groups and produce more shapely legs. Use heavier weights to build muscle. Cut back on your running to prevent further muscle loss, and up your daily protein intake – at least three portions of lean meat, fish, poultry, beans, lentils, dairy foods or other vegetarian protein sources

2 fat burning

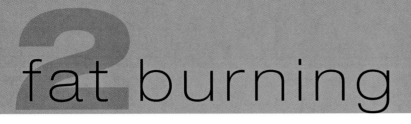

This six-week cardiovascular (CV) workout is designed to burn fat (and cellulite) and give you leaner, more contoured legs. It will also improve your aerobic fitness and heart health.

The first part of each workout is a cardiovascular (CV) routine designed to burn fat and improve your fitness. It consists of a warm-up, a CV section and a cool-down:

■ The **warm-up** raises your body temperature, prepares your body for more strenuous exercise and reduces injury risk.

■ The **CV section** should last for a minimum of 20 minutes. Each week you need to work a bit harder in order to continue making fitness gains. You can do any of the following: increase the number of times you work out per week (up to a maximum of five); increase your workout time (to a maximum of 60 minutes); increase the intensity, such as your speed or resistance of the machine; add more intervals (see page 11).

■ The **cool-down** allows your body temperature, muscles and circulatory system time to return to normal. If you stop too quickly, you may feel dizzy and faint.

cv workout guidelines

choose your activity

Any activity that uses the large muscle groups of the body and can be kept up for at least 20 minutes with your heart in the target heart rate range (see page 10) counts. Walking, running, elliptical training, rowing and cycling machines are good choices because they will tone your leg muscles as well as burn calories.

Remember, the higher the resistance, the greater the toning benefits, so raising the incline of the treadmill or increasing the resistance of the machine will help you in your quest for lovelier legs. Get comfortable with the programming features such as exercise time, distance goal, resistance level and any in-built workout programmes that simulate the conditions and terrain you're looking for (ask an instructor to help).

Try to vary your choice of CV activity so you challenge different muscle groups and don't get bored.

did you know?

Brisk walking for 45 minutes four times a week can result in fat loss of 40 kg (18 lb) over a year, according to top US cardiologist Dr James Rippe.

use target heart rate training

Make sure you are working out at a safe and effective level by using target heart rate training. This is a measure of how hard you are working. First of all you need to estimate your maximal heart rate (MHR) by subtracting your age from 220. For example, if you are 30, your MHR would be 220 – 30 = 190 beats per minute (bpm). Consult the Heart Rate Training Guide on page 10 to find out which zone you are training in. Each zone is basically a percentage of your MHR. Choose either the steady pace or interval CV workout, depending on your experience level.

Both workouts burn fat and develop your fitness – although the interval workout is more efficient.

monitor your heart rate

The best way to monitor your heart rate during your workout is by using a heart rate monitor, or by taking your pulse manually. At regular intervals count your heart rate at your wrist or neck for 10 seconds and multiply that number by six (which gives you your heart rate in beats per minute). Check to see which target heart rate (THR) zone you are in (see page 10).

use perceived exertion to monitor intensity

If you don't have a heart rate monitor and find it difficult to work out your heart rate manually, you can use perceived exertion (PE) instead of THR to monitor the intensity of your CV workout. This is a subjective rating of how hard you feel you are exercising (see page 11). It is a 10-point scale ranging from 1 (no effort at all) to 10 (maximum effort). This system correlates closely with THR, so if you're working out at PE level 6 you are exercising at about 60 per cent of your MHR.

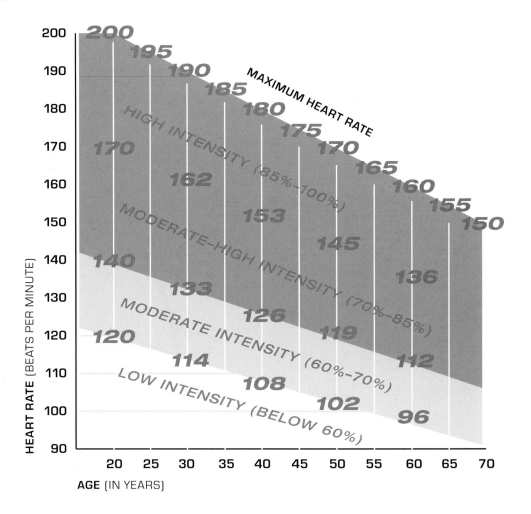

RATING OF PERCEIVED EXERTION (RPE)

At rest	1	Non-exercise HR
Light activity – sitting working	2	Non-exercise HR
Light activity – walking at leisurely pace	3	Non-exercise HR
Moderate activity – purposeful walking	4	Non-exercise HR
Moderate activity – brisk walking	5	Non-exercise HR
Somewhat hard activity – jogging	6	60% MHR
Hard activity – running, breathing harder	7	65–75% MHR
Very hard activity – running, conversation just possible	8	80% MHR
Very very hard activity – fast running, conversation difficult	9	85% MHR
Maximum effort – unable to speak	10	MHR

add intervals

Doing intervals – alternating short periods of high-intensity work with lower-intensity recovery periods – increases your calorie burn. It also helps you burn more calories afterwards. One US study found that interval training speeds up your metabolic rate up to 18 hours after your workout. It also gets you fitter and strengthens your heart and lungs more than training at a steady pace. However, intervals are only suitable for those with a good level of fitness to start with. Beginners should build up basic fitness with steady-pace exercise first.

Intervals can be applied to any mode of CV exercise – running, cycling, stationary bike, stepping machine, elliptical trainer or any other cardio machine. Intersperse faster bursts of activity (e.g. increase the speed or the resistance of the machine) with more moderate recovery periods.

getting started

Build up your pace or increase the resistance of your machine until you reach the required RPE. You should feel slightly breathless but comfortable (you should be able to talk in short sentences).

ELLIPTICAL TRAINER TECHNIQUE

- Maintain a good upright posture – spine in a neutral position and abdominals tight (check in a mirror).
- Keep your shoulders back and relaxed.
- Look forwards, not down at your feet. Your head should be level.
- Make sure your weight is evenly distributed and that your lower body supports most of your weight.
- Relax and maintain a comfortable smooth stride going through the normal range of motion.
- Avoid leaning too far forwards and hunching over the handles (which can be stressful for the back).

POWER WALKING TECHNIQUE

- Maintain a good posture by relaxing your shoulder muscles, keeping your shoulders down (not back) and ribcage slightly lifted. Look forwards rather than down.
- Walk tall and elegant, not tense and hunched.
- Hold your arms relaxed, close to the body, and hands cupped. Avoid swinging your arms across your body.
- As you walk, land on your heel and transfer your weight to the ball of your foot, rolling the foot in a smooth heel-to-toe movement.
- Stick to a comfortable stride length so your body is not forced to rotate through the hips.
- Keep your hips, knees and feet aligned – your feet should point directly forwards (this may feel awkward at first).
- Keep your body upright or angled just slightly forwards.
- Breathe deeply from the stomach.

RUNNING TECHNIQUE

- Keep your shoulders back and down in a relaxed, comfortable position.
- Try to keep your back straight and tall.
- Keep your torso upright and hold your abdominals tight.
- Use the power in your glutes (buttocks) and hamstrings (back of legs) to propel your body forwards.
- Land on your heels and roll through the whole foot – your toes should be last to leave the ground.
- Keep your feet close to the ground and take care not to bounce as you run.
- Keep your arms and hands loose and tension-free (don't clench your fists).
- Use a natural backwards and forwards swing with your arms – but don't exaggerate the action.
- Your feet, knees and hips should be in good alignment.
- Beginners tend to use very short strides, which stresses the knees – try to use a natural stride length.

ROWING TECHNIQUE

- Use the foot straps to keep your feet firmly in the machine, and keep your bottom firmly on the seat.
- Use your leg muscles to power the movement. Start the stroke (the 'drive') by pushing with your legs to drive you back along the machine (don't pull with your arms).
- Keep your arms extended in front of you until they reach the knees, then lean back slightly, pulling the handle towards your body.
- Bring the handle into your abdomen, not to your chest. Your elbows should be drawn past the body, not sticking out.
- At the end of the stroke, take care not to 'lock' your legs straight – keep the knees soft.
- You will know if you have poor technique, as you will hear the chain banging against the machine.

CYCLING TECHNIQUE

- Check your saddle height – in the downward phase of the cycling action, your leg should be extended but bent very slightly at the knee.
- Keep your neck and shoulders relaxed – avoid tensing your shoulders, and ensure there is a good distance between your ears and shoulders.
- Keep your arms straight but slightly bent at the elbows.
- Keep a firm but relaxed grip on the handles.
- Keep a neutral spine position in the saddle – keep as upright as possible and don't allow your back to slump forwards.
- Hold your stomach muscles tight – this will help to stabilise you.
- Your toes should point downwards slightly as you push down – this prevents tension in the calf muscles.
- Use toe clips if available – these allow you to use the muscles at the front and back of your legs to power the movement. Without clips, only the muscles at the front of the legs get worked.

STEADY PACE CV WORKOUT

Total exercise time = 30 minutes

Exercise time (minutes)	Stage	Intensity (THR)	Intensity (PE)
5	Warm-up	50%	5
20	Steady pace	60%	6
5	Cool-down	50%	5

INTERVAL CV WORKOUT

Total exercise time = 34 minutes

Exercise time (minutes)	Stage	Intensity (THR)	Intensity (PE)
5	Warm-up	50%	5
2	Interval	70%	7
2	Recovery	60%	6
2	Interval	70%	7
2	Recovery	60%	6
2	Interval	70%	7
2	Recovery	60%	6
2	Interval	70%	7
2	Recovery	60%	6
2	Interval	70%	7
2	Recovery	60%	6
2	Interval	70%	7
2	Recovery	60%	6
5	Cool down	50%	5

3 exercises

This six-week leg programme comprises a CV (fat-burning) workout followed by a sequence of toning exercises that target your legs. The six workouts increase in difficulty as the weeks progress. Each workout includes effective exercises that target every region of your legs – the front, outer, inner and back.

which fitness level?

If you're not currently exercising regularly, you should start at **level 1**, and aim to complete the suggested number of repetitions (reps). If you currently exercise at least three times a week, choose **level 2**. As you get accustomed to the exercises, you can gradually increase the number of repetitions or number of sets. But whichever level you are on, remember to focus on using good technique at all times.

workout rules

- Aim to complete each workout the suggested number of times per week.

- You may include other activities and sports on non-workout days but avoid working your legs intensely on these days.

- Allow at least two rest days per week to avoid over-training.

- If you experience discomfort, rest, then continue the workout.

- Each workout should take approximately 45–60 minutes to complete.

- For the toning exercises, make sure you perform each movement in a controlled manner, using a full range of motion and focusing on perfect form.

- If you find any of the exercises too difficult, adapt the movement so that it feels easier or substitute a similar exercise you are more familiar with until you develop enough strength.

- Focus on each movement – don't rush any exercise.

- Visualise your performance and your desired result – cut out a photo and stick it to your wall or fridge to keep you motivated.

week 1

the goal

The goal of the first week is to develop a good base of fitness and introduce you to an effective circuit of leg-toning exercises. In short, to get those legs working!

- Do the workout **two times** this week, resting at least one day in between workouts.
- Complete part 1 (CV exercise) followed by part 2 (toning exercises).
- Aim to complete the suggested time or repetitions (reps) – otherwise just do as many as you can.
- Perform all the exercises listed below (this is one circuit), repeating the circuit one more time.
- Rest for 30 seconds between exercises; rest for a minute after you finish a circuit.
- Perform each repetition with good technique (see 'Exercise Tips', pages 3–5).

part 1: cv exercise

day	workout
day 1	steady pace CV workout
day 2	interval CV workout

part 2: toning exercises

exercise	no. of circuits
Free-standing squat	2
Leg curls on the ball	2
Outer thigh raise	2
Inner thigh raise	2
One-legged calf raise	2

free-standing squat

target muscles: bottom, front thigh, back thigh, inner thigh, outer thigh

starting position

1. Stand with your feet shoulder-width apart (or slightly wider), toes angled out at 30 degrees.

movement

1. Keeping your head up and your back in neutral position, slowly lower yourself down until your thighs are parallel to the ground; it is not wise to go any further than this.

2. Keep your knees aligned over your feet, pointing in the direction of your toes.

3. Hold for a count of one, then return to the starting position.

Make it harder: Hold a pair of dumbbells by your sides.

TIPS

• You should maintain the natural curve in your back throughout the movement.

• Keep your tummy button gently pulled in towards the spine.

• Keep your eyes fixed on a point in front of you at about eye level.

• Make sure you do not bend forwards excessively as this will stress your lower back and reduce the emphasis on your legs.

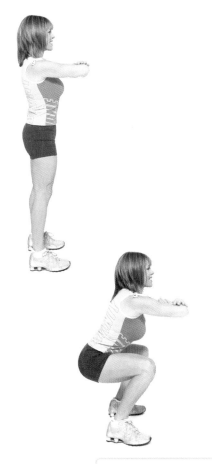

Level 1: 10–12 reps
Level 2: 15–20 reps

leg curls on the ball

target muscles: bottom, back of thigh

starting position

1. Lie on your back with your calves resting on an exercise ball and your hands by the sides of your thighs.

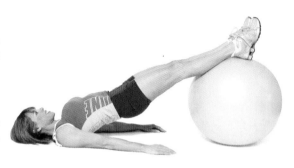

movement

1. Using your buttock muscles, lift your hips off the floor, rolling your vertebrae off the floor one by one.

2. You should make a diagonal line from your feet to your shoulders.

3. Push down into the ball through your feet and pull the ball in towards your bottom as far as you can. Keep your bottom lifted.

4. Slowly straighten your legs as you push the ball away from you. Do the number of repetitions listed below, then lower your hips slowly back to the starting position.

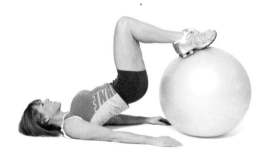

TIPS

- Keep the ball steady and moving in a straight line.
- Keep your hips lifted – they should not move up or down during the ball roll.
- Keep your neck and shoulders relaxed.

Level 1: 6–8 reps
Level 2: 8–10 reps

outer thigh raise

target muscles: outer thigh and hip

starting position

1. Lie on one side in a straight line.
2. Support your upper body on your forearm.
3. Place the other hand in front to steady yourself.

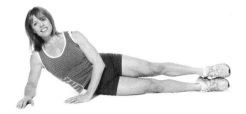

movement

1. Keeping your top leg straight and in line with your body, raise it up. Hold for a second then return to the starting position.
2. Do the number of repetitions listed below then turn on to your other side and repeat with your other leg.

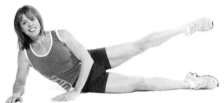

> **TIP**
>
> Make sure you keep your leg perfectly in line with your body – don't let it rotate to the front.

Level 1: 10–12 reps
Level 2: 15–20 reps

inner thigh raise

target muscles: inner thigh

starting position

1. Lie on one side in a straight line.
2. Support your upper body on your forearm.
3. Place the other hand in front to steady yourself.
4. Bend your top leg and place your foot on the floor just behind your lower leg.
5. Keep the lower leg straight.

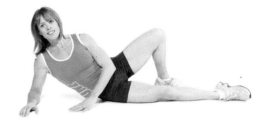

movement

1. Keeping your lower leg straight and your foot flexed, raise it as high as you can (a few centimetres would be fine). Hold for a second then return to the starting position.
2. Do the number of repetitions listed below then turn on to your other side and repeat with the other leg.

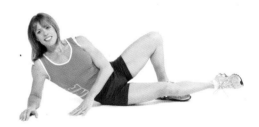

TIPS

- Keep the foot of your lower leg facing forwards and the inner part of the leg facing the ceiling.
- Keep your lower leg straight throughout the movement.

Level 1: 10–12 reps
Level 2: 15–20 reps

one-legged calf raise

target muscles: lower leg (calves)

starting position

1. Position the ball of your right foot on the edge of a step, allowing your heel to hang off the edge.

2. Hold on to a suitable support with the other hand to steady yourself.

movement

1. Rise as high as possible on the ball of your foot.

2. Hold this position for a count of two; then slowly lower your heel down as far as it will go.

3. Do the number of repetitions listed below, then perform the exercise with your left leg.

Make it harder: Hold a dumbbell in one hand.

TIPS

- Keep your exercising leg straight throughout the movement.
- Stretch your calf fully at the bottom of the movement – your heel should be lower than your toes.

Level 1: 10–12 reps
Level 2: 15–20 reps

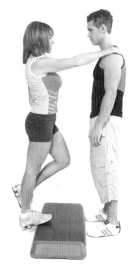

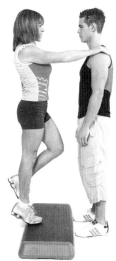

week 2

the goal

Your legs should be feeling great and ready to work a bit harder! Now that you've established the exercise habit, you can increase the workouts you do and add some new exercises to your routine. You'll continue with the fat-burning CV exercise, followed by two circuits of exercises to firm up those thighs.

- Do the workout **three times** this week, resting at least one day between workouts.
- Complete part 1 (CV exercise) followed by part 2 (toning exercises).
- Aim to complete the suggested time or repetitions (reps) – otherwise just do as many as you can.
- Perform all the exercises listed below (this is one circuit), repeating the circuit one more time.
- Rest for 30 seconds between exercises; rest for a minute after you finish a circuit.
- Perform each repetition with good technique (see 'Exercise Tips', pages 3–5).

part 1: **cv exercise**

day	workout
day 1	steady pace
day 2	interval CV workout
day 3	steady pace CV workout

part 2: **toning exercises**

exercise	no. of circuits
Squat with the ball	2
Inner thigh toner	2
Front lunge	2
Seated leg curl or leg curls on the ball (page 20)*	2
Standing calf raise	2

* Depending on availability of equipment

squat with the ball

target muscles: bottom, front of thigh, back of thigh, inner thigh

starting position

1. Put an exercise ball just behind you against a wall. Stand with your lower back firmly against it.
2. Position your feet shoulder-width apart, slightly further forward than your shoulders.
3. Cross your arms over your chest.

movement

1. Slowly bend your knees to roll the ball down the wall. Lower until your thighs are parallel to the ground, maintaining the normal arch in your spine.
2. Pressing through your heels, raise yourself back up again as you straighten your legs.

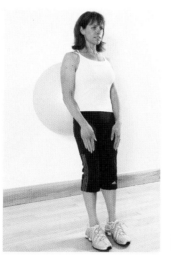
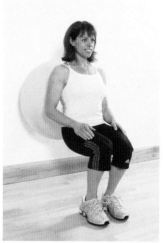

TIPS

- Keep the normal curve in your spine by contracting your abdominals.
- Look directly ahead.

Level 1: 10–12 reps
Level 2: 15–20 reps

inner thigh toner

target muscles: inner thigh

starting position

1. Lie on your back with your legs raised and an exercise ball between your bent knees.

movement

1. Squeeze the ball with your inner thighs and knees.
2. Hold for a second, then release and do the number of repetitions listed below.

Make it harder:

- *Hold the squeeze for several seconds.*
- *Place the ball between your ankles and calves, keeping your knees slightly bent.*

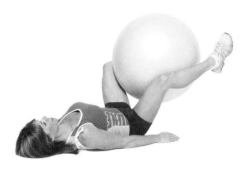

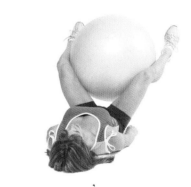

TIPS

- You may wish to hold the ball with your hands to keep it steady.
- Draw your navel towards your spine to prevent your back arching.

Level 1: 8–10 reps
Level 2: 12–15 reps

front lunge

target muscles: front of thigh, back of thigh, bottom

starting position

1. Stand with your feet shoulder-width apart, toes pointing forwards

movement

1. Take an exaggerated step forwards with your right leg, bending the knee and lowering your hips. Lower yourself until your right thigh is parallel to the floor and your knee is at an angle of 90 degrees. Your left leg should be about 10–15 cm above the floor. Hold for a second.

2. Push hard with your right leg to return to the starting position.

3. Carry out the number of repetitions listed below, then perform the movement with the left leg leading.

Make it harder: Hold a pair of dumbbells.

TIPS

- Keep your front knee positioned directly over your ankle – do not allow it to extend further forwards as this can cause strain to the knee.

- Keep your body erect throughout the movement – do not lean forwards.

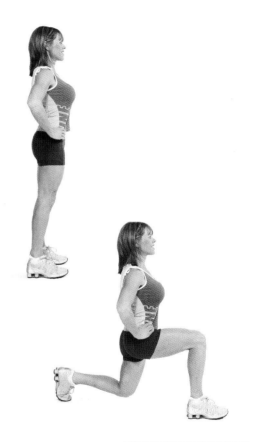

Level 1: 8–10 reps
Level 2: 12–15 reps

seated leg curl

target muscles: back of thigh

starting position

1. Sit down in the leg curl machine and place your heels over the roller pads.
2. Adjust the machine if necessary so your knees are just off the end of the bench and your thighs are fully supported.
3. Hold on to the handgrips or the edge of the bench for support.

movement

1. Bend your knees, bringing your heels towards your backside.
2. Hold for a count of two, then slowly return to the starting position.

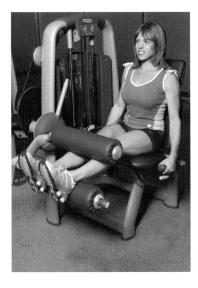
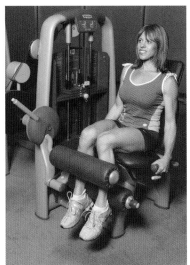

TIP

If a leg curl machine is not available, perform leg curls on the ball (page 20) instead.

Level 1: 8–10 reps
Level 2: 12–15 reps

standing calf raise

target muscles: lower leg (calves)

starting position

1. Position the balls of your feet on a step so that your heels hang over the edge. You can support yourself on your training partner if necessary.

movement

1. Rise on your toes as high as possible.
2. Hold the position for a count of two, then slowly lower your heels down as far as they will go.

Make it harder: Perform this exercise on a calf raise or Smith machine; or place a light barbell across your shoulders.

TIPS

- Keep your legs straight (but not locked) throughout the movement.
- Stretch your calves fully at the bottom of the movement – your heels should be lower than your toes.

Level 1: 10–12 reps
Level 2: 15–20 reps

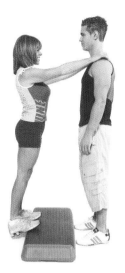

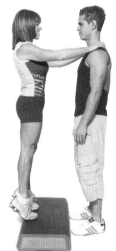

week 3

This week, you'll be progressing from a circuit routine to a sets-based workout. This means you'll be performing a number of sets of each exercise, separated by a short rest, before moving on to the next exercise. You'll have to work a little harder, but you'll be well on your way to firmer thighs by the end of this week.

■ Do the workout **three times** this week, resting at least one day between workouts.

■ Complete part 1 (CV exercise) followed by part 2 (toning exercises).

■ Aim to complete the suggested time or repetitions (reps) – otherwise just do as many as you can.

■ Rest for 30 seconds between each set.

■ After completing the suggested number of sets for each exercise, rest for a minute before moving on to the next exercise.

■ Perform each repetition with good technique (see 'Exercise Tips', pages 3–5).

part 1: cv exercise

day	workout
day 1	interval CV workout
day 2	steady pace CV workout
day 3	interval CV workout

part 2: toning exercises

exercise	sets
Reverse lunge	2 – 3
Dumbbell step-ups	2 – 3
Outer and inner thigh shaper	2 – 3
Calf press or one-legged calf raise (page 23)*	2 – 3

* Depending on availability of equipment

reverse lunge

target muscles: back of thigh, front of thigh, bottom

starting position

1. Stand with your feet shoulder-width apart, toes pointing forwards.

movement

1. Take a large step backwards with your right leg, bending your left leg and lowering your hips. Keep your trunk upright.

2. Lower yourself into a one-legged squat position on your left leg until your left thigh is parallel to the floor. Your left knee should be at an angle of 90 degrees. Hold for a second, then push hard through your left leg to return to the starting position. Don't push through your right (back) leg.

3. Perform the number of repetitions listed below, then repeat with the left leg leading.

Make it harder: Hold a pair of dumbbells. Alternatively, perform the movement with a Smith machine. Stand directly under the bar of the Smith machine so that it rests fairly low across your upper back while allowing you to maintain an upright posture. Hold the bar and lift it from the rack, unlocking the safety catches. Perform the movement as above.

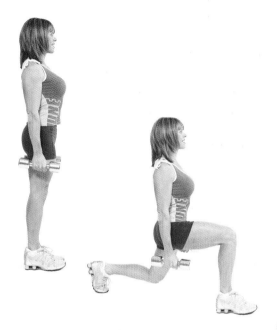

TIPS

• Keep your body erect throughout the movement – do not lean forwards.

• Make sure you step back far enough so that when you lower your body, the knee of your front leg doesn't pass your toes. In the bottom position your shin should be vertical.

Level 1: 2 sets 8–10 reps
Level 2: 3 sets 12–15 reps

dumbbell step-ups

target muscles: front of thigh, back of thigh, bottom

starting position

1. Stand facing a step, holding a pair of dumbbells.

movement

1. Step onto the step with one foot then lift your other foot up to the step.
2. Step down with the second leg, then the first.
3. Repeat with the second leg leading.

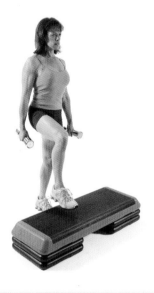

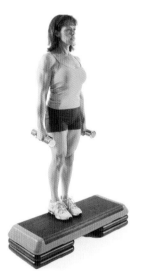

TIPS

- Do not allow your body to lean forwards while stepping up.
- Make sure your foot is securely on the step when you step up.

Make it harder: Increase the height of the step.

Level 1: 2 sets 10–12 reps
Level 2: 3 sets 15–20 reps

outer and inner thigh shaper

target muscles: outer thigh and inner thigh

starting position

1. Lie on your right side in a straight line.
2. Position an exercise ball between your feet.
3. Extend your lower arm out to cushion your head and place the other hand in front to steady yourself.

movement

1. Squeeze the ball between your feet, pushing down with your top leg and up with your bottom leg.
2. Hold for a second, then release and carry out the number of repetitions listed below.
3. Repeat the movement lying on your left side.

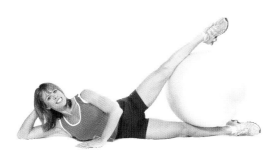 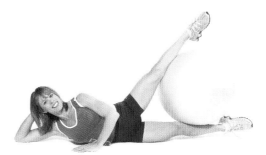

TIPS

• Try to lift your waist from the floor – don't let it drop back down.
• Pull your navel in towards your spine.

Level 1: 2 sets 8–10 reps
Level 2: 3 sets 12–15 reps

calf press

target muscles: lower leg (calves)

starting position

1. Position yourself in a leg press machine.

2. Place the balls of your feet on the bottom of the platform with your heels hanging over the edge. Your legs should be fully extended and feet hip-width apart.

3. Release the safety catch.

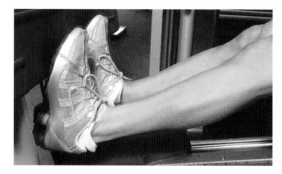

movement

1. Press the platform away from you as far as possible.

2. Hold the fully contracted position for a count of two.

3. Slowly lower your heels down as far as they will go.

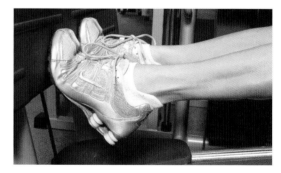

TIPS

- Stretch your calves fully at the bottom of the movement – your heels should be lower than your toes.

- Keep your legs straight (not locked) throughout the movement.

- If a leg press machine is not available, perform one-legged calf raise (page 23) instead.

Level 1: 2 sets 10–12 reps
Level 2: 3 sets 15–20 reps

week 4

You'll continue to perform two to three sets of each exercise but will now be reducing the rest time between sets. Try to push yourself harder by doing a few more repetitions of each exercise.

- Do the workout **three times** this week, resting at least one day between workouts.
- Complete part 1 (CV exercise) followed by part 2 (toning exercises).
- Aim to complete the suggested time or repetitions (reps) – otherwise just do as many as you can.
- Rest for 20 seconds between each set.
- After completing the suggested number of sets for each exercise, rest for 30–45 seconds before moving on to the next exercise.
- Perform each repetition with good technique (see 'Exercise Tips', pages 3–5).

part 1: cv exercise

day	workout
day 1	steady pace CV workout
day 2	interval CV workout
day 3	steady pace CV workout

part 2: toning exercises

exercise	sets
Split squat	2–3
Leg press or free-standing squat (page 19)*	2–3
Leg extension on all fours	2–3
Seated calf raise or standing calf raise (page 29)*	2–3

* Depending on availability of equipment

split squat

target muscles: bottom, back of thigh, front of thigh, inner thigh, outer thigh

starting position

1. Take a step forwards with your right leg and a step back with your left. Your left heel will lift off the floor.

movement

1. Drop your body downwards, bending your right knee to 90 degrees, bringing your rear knee to a point just above the floor.

2. Push back up through the front heel into a standing split squat.

3. Carry out the number of repetitions listed below, then switch legs to complete the set.

Make it harder:

■ *Hold a pair of dumbbells or perform the movement with a Smith machine, positioning the bar across your upper back.*

■ *Put your rear foot on a block or step about 15 cm high. This increases the range of motion and you will feel a greater stretch in the quadriceps of the rear leg.*

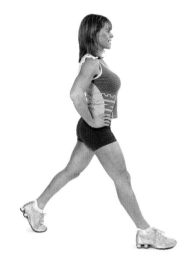

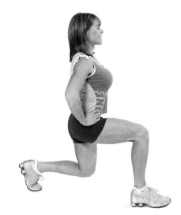

TIPS

• When descending, think about dropping your hips straight down so you avoid bending forwards.

• Keep your front knee positioned directly over your ankle – do not allow it to extend further forwards.

Level 1: 2 sets 10–12 reps
Level 2: 3 sets 15–20 reps

leg press

target muscles: bottom, front of thigh, back of thigh

starting position

1. Sit into the base of the leg press machine with your back firmly against the padding.
2. Position your feet parallel and hip-width apart on the platform.
3. Release the safety bars and extend your legs.

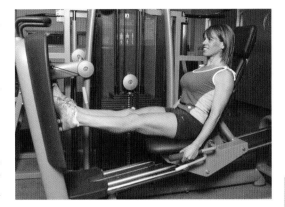

movement

1. Slowly bend your legs and lower the platform in a controlled fashion until your knees almost touch your chest. Hold for a second.
2. Return the platform to the starting position, pushing hard through your heels.
3. Carry out the number of repetitions listed below.

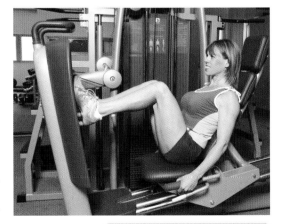

TIPS

- Keep your back in full contact with the base; do not allow your lower spine to curl up as you lower the platform.
- Keep your knees in line with your toes.
- If a leg press machine is not available, perform the free-standing squat (page 19) instead.

Level 1: 2 sets 10–12 reps
Level 2: 3 sets 15–20 reps

leg extension on all fours

target muscles: bottom, back of thigh, inner thigh, lower back

starting position

1. Position yourself on all fours.

2. Ensure your back is flat and parallel to the floor and your knees are directly under your hips.

movement

1. Bring your right knee in towards your chest, then extend your right leg straight out behind you. Aim to form a straight line from your head to your foot, parallel to the floor.

2. Bring your right knee in towards your chest and repeat as listed below.

3. Do the movement with your left leg for the number of repetitions listed below.

1 2 3 4

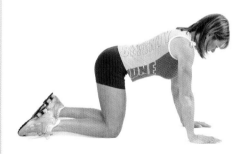 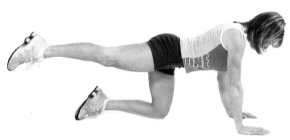

TIPS

• Avoid rotating your hips as you push your leg out behind – keep them square to the floor.

• Keep your back flat throughout the movement.

Level 1: 2 sets 10–12 reps
Level 2: 3 sets 15–20 reps

seated calf raise

target muscles: lower leg (calves)

starting position

1. Sit on a bench in front of a step and place a barbell across your lower thighs. Alternatively, position yourself on a seated calf-raise machine, adjusting the pad height to fit snugly over your lower thighs.

2. Place the balls of your feet on the step or platform, making sure they are directly below your knees.

movement

1. Rise up on to the balls of your feet and hold for at least 2 seconds.

2. Slowly lower your heels until they are as far below the balls of your feet as possible.

3. Carry out the number of repetitions listed below.

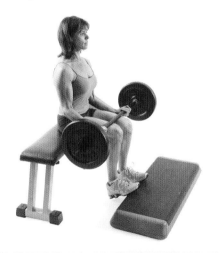
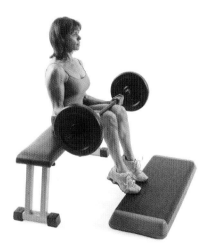

TIP

Make sure you perform this exercise through a full range of movement. If the correct apparatus is not available, perform the standing calf raise (page 29) instead.

Level 1: 2 sets 10–12 reps
Level 2: 3 sets 15–20 reps

week 5

To increase the toning benefits, you'll progress from straight sets to supersets this week. This means you'll perform the first exercise then, without resting, immediately move on to the second exercise. You'll then take a short rest before repeating the superset. Easy? Well, if you want great legs, you'll have to work hard.

■ Do the workout **three times** this week, resting at least one day between workouts.

■ Complete part 1 (CV exercise) followed by part 2 (toning exercises).

■ Aim to complete the repetitions (reps) – otherwise just do as many as you can.

■ Perform the two exercises in the first superset without taking a rest. Then rest for a minute and repeat once.

■ Next, perform the second superset without taking a rest. Rest for a minute then repeat once.

■ Perform each repetition with good technique (see 'Exercise Tips', pages 3–5).

part 1: cv exercise

day	workout
day 1	interval CV workout
day 2	steady pace CV workout
day 3	interval CV workout

part 2: **toning exercises**

exercise	sets
Superset 1	
Squat with the ball (see page 25 but complete 12–15 reps for level 1; 15–20 reps for level 2)	2
Reverse lunge with dumbbells	2
Superset 2	
Leg extension or dumbbell step-ups (page 32)*	2
Seated leg curl (page 28) or leg curls on the ball (page 20)*	2
One-legged calf raise (page 23)	2–3

* Depending on availability of equipment

reverse lunge with dumbbells

target muscles: back of thigh, front of thigh, bottom

starting position

1. Stand with your feet shoulder-width apart, toes pointing forwards.

2. Hold a pair of dumbbells by your sides.

movement

1. Take a large step backwards with your left leg, bending your right leg and lowering your hips. Keep your trunk upright.

2. Lower yourself into a one-legged squat position on your right leg until your right thigh is parallel to the floor. Your right knee should be at an angle of 90 degrees. Hold for a second, then push hard through your right leg to return to the starting position. Don't push through your left (back) leg.

3. Perform the number of repetitions listed below, then repeat with the right leg leading.

TIPS

- Keep your body erect throughout the movement – do not lean forwards.
- Make sure you step back far enough so the knee of your front leg doesn't pass your toes when you lower your body. In the bottom position your shin should be vertical.

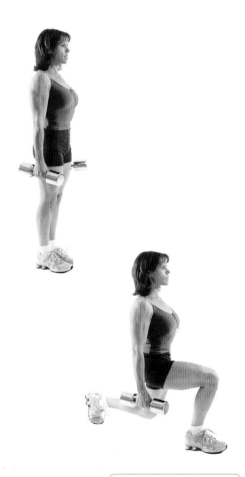

Level 1: 8–10 reps
Level 2: 12–15 reps

1 2 3 4 5

leg extension

target muscles: front of thigh

starting position

1. Sit on the leg extension machine, adjusting it so that the backs of your thighs are fully supported on the seat.

2. Hook your feet under the foot pads. The pads should rest on the lowest part of your shins, just above your ankles.

3. Hold on to the sides of the seat or the handles on the sides of the machine to prevent your hips lifting as you perform the exercise.

movement

1. Straighten your legs to full extension, keeping your thighs and backside fully in contact with the bench.

2. Hold this fully contracted position for a count of two, then slowly return to the starting point.

TIPS

- Do not allow your hips to rise off the seat.
- Try to 'resist' the weight as you lower your legs back to the starting point – avoid letting the weight swing your legs back.
- If a leg extension machine is not available, perform dumbell step-ups (page 32) instead.

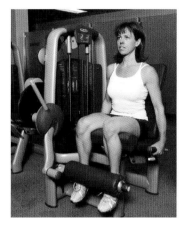

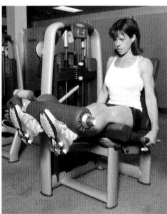

Level 1: 8–10 reps
Level 2: 12–15 reps

week 6

This week further challenges your fitness and strength by introducing two power movements: the straddle box jump and the switch split jump. These exercises develop speed and explosive power without increasing muscle size. Performed as part of a superset, they will challenge your muscles, resulting in further toning benefits.

■ Do the workout **three times** this week, resting at least one day between workouts.

■ Complete part 1 (CV exercise) followed by part 2 (toning exercises).

■ Aim to complete the repetitions (reps) – otherwise just do as many as you can.

■ Perform the two exercises in the first superset without taking a rest. Then rest for a minute and repeat once.

■ Next, perform the second superset without taking a rest. Rest for a minute then repeat once.

■ Perform each repetition with good technique (see 'Exercise Tips', pages 3–5).

part 1: cv exercise

day	workout
day 1	steady pace CV workout
day 2	interval CV workout
day 3	steady pace CV workout

part 2: **toning exercises**

exercise	sets
Superset 1	
Walking lunge	2
Straddle box jump	2
Superset 2	
Straight-leg dead lift	2
Switch split jump	2
Standing calf raise	
(page 29)	2–3

walking lunge

target muscles: front of thigh, back of thigh, bottom

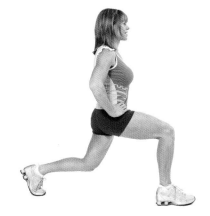

starting position

1. Stand with your feet shoulder-width apart, toes pointing forwards. Make sure you have enough space in front of you to do your target number of steps.

movement

1. Take an exaggerated step forwards with your right leg, bending the knee and lowering your hips. Lower yourself until your right thigh is parallel to the floor and your knee is at an angle of 90 degrees. Your left leg should be about 10–15 cm above the floor. Hold for a second.

2. Push hard with your right leg as you straighten up, bring your left leg through then take an exaggerated step forwards with your left leg.

3. Carry out the number of repetitions listed below.

Make it harder: Hold a pair of dumbbells.

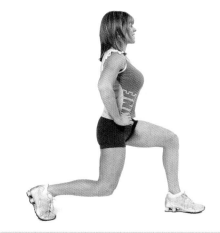

TIPS

• Keep your front knee positioned directly over your ankle – do not allow it to extend further forwards as this can cause strain to the knee.

• Keep your body erect throughout the movement – do not lean forwards.

Level 1: 6–8 reps (12–16 total steps)
Level 2: 10–12 reps (20–24 total steps)

123456

straddle box jump

target muscles: front of thigh, inner thigh, outer thigh

starting position

1. Stand astride a sturdy low gym box or aerobics step.

movement

1. Jump straight up above the box. Land with both feet on top of the box, making sure you bend your knees for a soft landing.

2. Either jump-drop both feet back to the floor or step down with one foot, then the other.

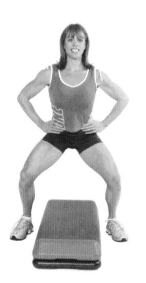

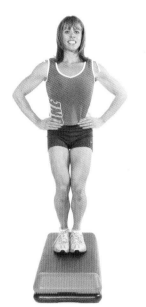

Make it harder: Use a higher box or step. This makes it more difficult as you need to jump higher.

Level 1: 6–8 reps
Level 2: 10–12 reps

straight-leg dead lift

target muscles: back of thigh, bottom

starting position

1. Grasp a bar or pair of dumbbells with your hands slightly wider than shoulder-width apart, using an overhand grip.

2. Stand up straight, looking directly ahead.

movement

1. Keeping your back flat and with a slight bend in your knees, bend forwards from the hips until your back is parallel to the ground. You should feel a stretch in your hamstrings and gluteals.

2. As you bend forwards, your hips and gluteals should move backwards and your body should be centred through your heels.

3. Hold for a second then return to the erect starting position.

This exercise is suitable only for advanced exercisers, as it requires a high degree of technical skill. Avoid if you have back problems. You can substitute Leg Curls on the Ball (page 20) or Seated Leg Curl (page 28).

Level 1: 8–10 reps
Level 2: 12–15 reps

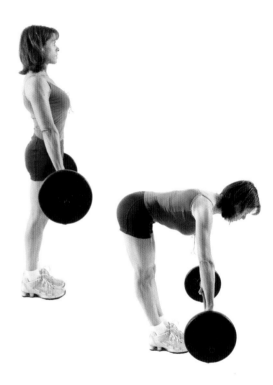

TIPS

• Hinge at the hips and keep your back flat – rounding your back will increase the risk of injury.

• Do not lower the bar or dumbbells too far. They should be hanging at arms' length below you, at about knee level.

switch split jump

target muscles: front of thigh, hamstrings, bottom

starting position

1. Stand with your feet together.
2. Keeping your head up and back straight, take a small step forwards with your right foot.
3. Bend both your knees, making sure your right knee doesn't pass over your toes.

movement

1. Jump up, straightening your legs and switching position with your feet.
2. Land in the starting position with your left foot forwards and repeat.

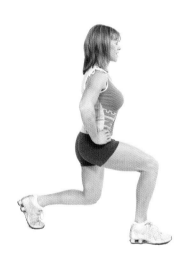
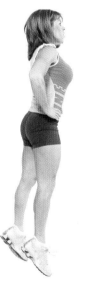
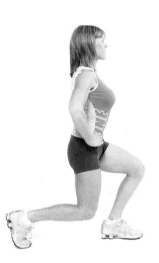

TIPS

- Keep your back straight throughout the movement – don't lean forwards when landing.
- Try doing this exercise in front of a mirror.

Level 1: 6–8 reps
Level 2: 10–12 reps

the stretches

Stretching at the end of each workout will help improve your flexibility and posture, and make your muscles look leaner and longer. Make sure you focus on your form and technique.

You should only stretch when your body is warm and the muscle is receiving an increased blood flow. Stretching a cold muscle increases the risk of injury and reduces the effectiveness of the stretch. Here are some basic guidelines:

- Ideally, stretching should be done after a workout and also between sets.
- Alternatively, stretch between workouts as a separate session but only after a thorough warm-up – 5–10 minutes of some light aerobic activity.
- Perform static stretches and avoid bouncing.
- Gradually ease into position, focusing all the time on relaxing the muscle.
- Stretch only as far as is comfortable, then hold that position. As the muscle relaxes, ease further into the stretch, gradually increasing the range of motion.
- Never hold your breath. Exhale and relax as you go into the stretch and then breathe normally.
- Never go past the point of discomfort or pain. You could pull or tear the muscle or tendon.
- Stretches performed at the end of a workout, or during a separate session, should be held for 30 seconds or more to allow stretching in the connective tissue and muscle.
- Release from the stretch slowly.

standing front thigh stretch

Hold on to a sturdy support. Bend one leg up behind you and hold your ankle. Keeping your thighs level and knees close together, push your hips forwards until you feel a good stretch. Repeat on the other side.

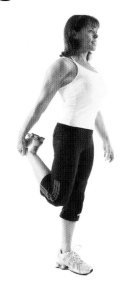

seated inner thigh stretch

Sit on the floor and place the soles of your feet together. Hold on to your ankles and press your thighs down using your elbows. Keep your back straight.

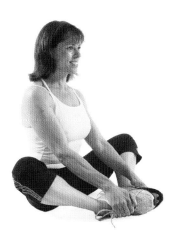

standing inner thigh stretch

Stand with your legs approximately double shoulder-width apart. With your left foot pointing forwards and your right foot turned to the side, bend your right knee until it forms a 90-degree angle directly over your foot. Hold and repeat on the other side.

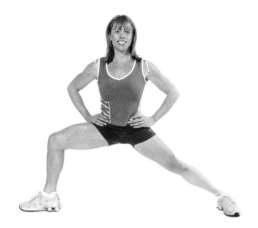

hamstring stretch

Sit on the floor with one leg extended and the other leg bent. Keeping your back straight and flat, hinge forwards from the hips. Reach down towards your foot. Flexing your foot will increase the stretch on the calf. Repeat on the other side.

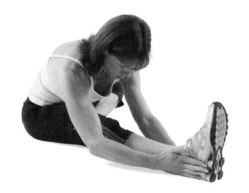

hip flexor stretch

From a kneeling position, take a large step forwards so that your knee makes a 90-degree angle and is directly over your foot. Keep your body upright and press your rear hip forwards, keeping it square. Repeat on the other side.

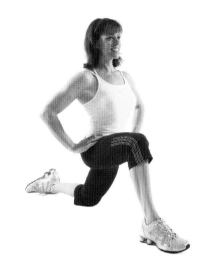

hip and outer thigh stretch

Sit on the floor and cross one foot over your straight leg. Place your elbow on the outside of the bent knee and slowly look over your shoulder on the side of the bent leg. Keep your opposite arm behind your hips for stability. Apply pressure to the knee with your elbow. Repeat on the other side.

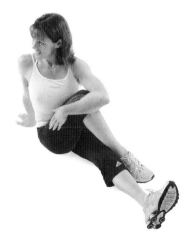

calf stretch

From a standing position, take an exaggerated step forwards, keeping your rear leg straight. Hold on to a wall for support if you wish. Your front knee should be at an angle of 90 degrees and positioned over your foot. Lean forwards slightly so that your rear leg and body make a continuous line, then repeat with the other leg.

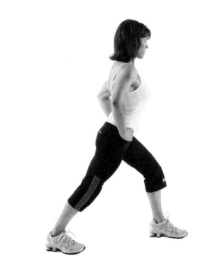

seesaw

Stand upright with your feet hip-width apart and arms by your sides. Slide your left leg behind you as you hinge forwards at the hip so that your upper body and left leg are parallel to the floor. Lift your arms so they are parallel to the floor. Aim to achieve a straight line from your fingers to your toes.

Draw your navel in towards your spine and visualise lengthening your whole body from your fingers to your feet.

At first you may only be able to balance at an angle to the floor – this is fine, provided you maintain a straight line from fingers to toes.

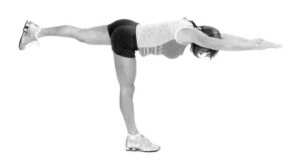

shoulder bridge

Lie on your back with your calves resting on an exercise ball and your hands by the sides of your thighs. Using your buttock muscles, lift your hips off the floor, rolling your vertebrae off the floor one by one. You should make a diagonal line from your feet to your shoulders. Hold for a second, pushing your heels down into the ball and lengthening your spine. Then slowly lower your hips to the floor, laying the vertebrae down one by one.

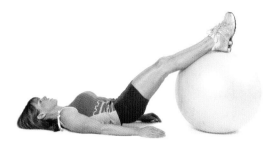

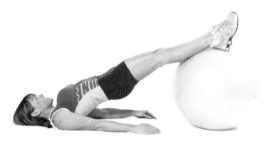

4 workout logs

Use the workout logs in this chapter to record your progress throughout the six-week workout programme. You can choose which days of the week suit you best for your workouts, as long as you take the same number of rest days between them. The days given below are guidelines only.

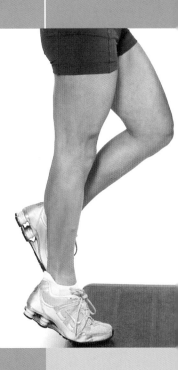

	day	workout	exercise	goal reps	actual reps
week 1	Monday	Steady pace CV workout			
		Leg toning exercises	Free-standing squat	10–12 or 15–20	Circuit 1: Circuit 2:
			Leg curls on the ball	6–8 or 8–10	Circuit 1: Circuit 2:
			Outer thigh raise	10–12 or 15–20	Circuit 1: Circuit 2:
			Inner thigh raise	10–12 or 15–20	Circuit 1: Circuit 2:
			One-legged calf raise	10–12 or 15–20	Circuit 1: Circuit 2:
	Tuesday	Rest day			
	Wednesday	Rest day			
	Thursday	Interval CV workout			
		Leg toning exercises	Free-standing squat	10–12 or 15–20	Circuit 1: Circuit 2:
			Leg curls on the ball	6–8 or 8–10	Circuit 1: Circuit 2:
			Outer thigh raise	10–12 or 15–20	Circuit 1: Circuit 2:
			Inner thigh raise	10–12 or 15–20	Circuit 1: Circuit 2:
			One-legged calf raise	10–12 or 15–20	Circuit 1: Circuit 2:
	Friday	Rest day			
	Saturday	Rest day			
	Sunday	Rest day			

week 2	day	workout	exercise	goal reps	actual reps
	Monday	Interval CV workout			
		Leg toning workout	Squat with the ball	10 – 12 or 15 – 20	Circuit 1: Circuit 2:
			Inner thigh toner	8 – 10 or 12 – 15	Circuit 1: Circuit 2:
			Front lunge	8 – 10 or 12 – 15	Circuit 1: Circuit 2:
			Seated leg curl or Leg curls on the ball	8 – 10 or 12 – 15 6 – 8 or 8 – 10	Circuit 1: Circuit 2:
			Standing calf raise	10 – 12 or 15 – 20	Circuit 1: Circuit 2:
	Tuesday	Rest day			
	Wednesday	Steady pace CV workout			
		Leg toning workout	Squat with the ball	10 – 12 or 15 – 20	Circuit 1: Circuit 2:
			Inner thigh toner	8 – 10 or 12 – 15	Circuit 1: Circuit 2:
			Front lunge	8 – 10 or 12 – 15	Circuit 1: Circuit 2:
			Seated leg curl or Leg curls on the ball	8 – 10 or 12 – 15 6 – 8 or 8 – 10	Circuit 1: Circuit 2:
			Standing calf raise	10 – 12 or 15 – 20	Circuit 1: Circuit 2:
	Thursday	Rest day			

Friday	Interval CV workout			
	Leg toning workout	Squat with the ball	10–12 or 15–20	Circuit 1: Circuit 2:
		Inner thigh toner	8–10 or 12–15	Circuit 1: Circuit 2:
		Front lunge	8–10 or 12–15	Circuit 1: Circuit 2:
		Seated leg curl or Leg curls on the ball	8–10 or 12–15 6–8 or 8–10	Circuit 1: Circuit 2:
		Standing calf raise	10–12 or 15–20	Circuit 1: Circuit 2:
Saturday	Rest day			
Sunday	Rest day			

	day	workout	exercise	goal reps	actual reps
week 3	Monday	Steady pace CV workout			
		Leg toning workout	Reverse lunge	8–10 or 12–15	Set 1: Set 2: Set 3:
			Dumbbell step-ups	10–12 or 15–20	Set 1: Set 2: Set 3:
			Outer and inner thigh shaper	8–10 or 12–15	Set 1: Set 2: Set 3:
			Calf press or One-legged calf raise	10–12 or 15–20 10–12 or 15–20	Set 1: Set 2: Set 3:
	Tuesday	Rest day			
	Wednesday	Interval CV workout			
		Leg toning workout	Reverse lunge	8–10 or 12–15	Set 1: Set 2: Set 3:
			Dumbbell step-ups	10–12 or 15–20	Set 1: Set 2: Set 3:
			Outer and inner thigh shaper	8–10 or 12–15	Set 1: Set 2: Set 3:
			Calf press or One-legged calf raise	10–12 or 15–20 10–12 or 15–20	Set 1: Set 2: Set 3:
	Thursday	Rest day			

	Friday	Steady pace CV workout			
		Leg toning workout	Reverse lunge workout	8 – 10 or 12 – 15	Set 1: Set 2: Set 3:
			Dumbbell step-ups	10 – 12 or 15 – 20	Set 1: Set 2: Set 3:
			Outer and inner thigh shaper	8 – 10 or 12 – 15	Set 1: Set 2: Set 3:
			Calf press or One-legged calf raise	10 – 12 or 15 – 20 10 – 12 or 15 – 20	Set 1: Set 2: Set 3:
	Saturday	Rest day			
	Sunday	Rest day			

	day	workout	exercise	goal reps	actual reps
week 4	Monday	Interval CV workout			
		Leg toning workout	Split squat	10–12 or 15–20	Set 1: Set 2: Set 3:
			Leg press or Free-standing squat	10–12 or 15–20 10–12 or 15–20	Set 1: Set 2: Set 3:
			Leg extension on all fours	10–12 or 15–20	Set 1: Set 2: Set 3:
			Seated calf raise or Standing calf raise	10–12 or 15–20 10–12 or 15–20	Set 1: Set 2: Set 3:
	Tuesday	Rest day			
	Wednesday	Steady pace CV workout			
		Leg toning workout	Split squat	10–12 or 15–20	Set 1: Set 2: Set 3:
			Leg press or Free-standing squat	10–12 or 15–20 10–12 or 15–20	Set 1: Set 2: Set 3:
			Leg extension on all fours	10–12 or 15–20	Set 1: Set 2: Set 3:
			Seated calf raise or Standing calf raise	10–12 or 15–20 10–12 or 15–20	Set 1: Set 2: Set 3:
	Thursday	Rest day			

Friday	Interval CV workout			
	Leg toning workout	Split squat workout	10–12 or 15–20	Set 1: Set 2: Set 3:
		Leg press or Free-standing squat	10–12 or 15–20 10–12 or 15–20	Set 1: Set 2: Set 3:
		Leg extension on all fours	10–12 or 15–20	Set 1: Set 2: Set 3:
		Seated calf raise or Standing calf raise	10–12 or 15–20 10–12 or 15–20	Set 1: Set 2: Set 3:
Saturday	Rest day			
Sunday	Rest day			

	day	workout	exercise	goal reps	actual reps
week 5	Monday	Steady pace CV workout			
		Leg toning workout	**Superset 1**		
			Squat with the ball	12 – 15 or 15 – 20	Set 1: Set 2:
			Reverse lunge with dumbbells	8 – 10 or 12 – 15	Set 1: Set 2:
			Superset 2		
			Leg extension or or Dumbbell step-ups	8 – 10 or 12 – 15 10 – 12 or 15 – 20	Set 1: Set 2:
			Seated leg curl or Leg curls on the ball	8 – 10 or 12 – 15 6 – 8 or 8 – 10	Set 1: Set 2:
			One-legged calf raise	10 – 12 or 15 – 20	Set 1: Set 2: Set 3:
	Tuesday	Rest day			
	Wednesday	Interval CV workout			
		Leg toning workout	**Superset 1**		
			Squat with the ball	12 – 15 or 15 – 20	Set 1: Set 2:
			Reverse lunge with dumbbells	8 – 10 or 12 – 15	Set 1: Set 2:

		Superset 2		
		Leg extension or Dumbbell step-ups	8 – 10 or 12 – 15 10 – 12 or 15 – 20	Set 1: Set 2:
		Seated leg curl or Leg curls on the ball	8 – 10 or 12 – 15 6 – 8 or 8 – 10	Set 1: Set 2:
		One-legged calf raise	10 – 12 or 15 – 20	Set 1: Set 2: Set 3:
Thursday	Rest day			
Friday	Steady pace CV workout			
	Leg toning workout	**Superset 1**		
		Squat with the ball	12 – 15 or 15 – 20	Set 1: Set 2: Set 3:
		Reverse lunge with dumbbells	8 – 10 or 12 – 15	Set 1: Set 2:
		Superset 2		
		Leg extension or Dumbbell step-ups	8 – 10 or 12 – 15 10 – 12 or 15 – 20	Set 1: Set 2:
		Seated leg curl or Legs curls on the ball	8 – 10 or 12 – 15 6 – 8 or 8 – 10	Set 1: Set 2:
		One-legged calf raise	10 – 12 or 15 – 20	Set 1: Set 2: Set 3:
Saturday	Rest day			
Sunday	Rest day			

	day	workout	exercise	goal reps	actual reps
week 6	Monday	Interval CV workout			
		Leg toning workout	**Superset 1**		
			Walking lunge	6–8 or 10–12	Set 1: Set 2:
			Straddle box jump	6–8 or 10–12	Set 1: Set 2:
			Superset 2		
			Straight-leg dead lift	8–10 or 12–15	Set 1: Set 2:
			Switch split jump	6–8 or 10–12	Set 1: Set 2:
			Standing calf raise	10–12 or 15–20	Set 1: Set 2: Set 3:
	Tuesday	Rest day			
	Wednesday	Steady pace CV workout			
		Leg toning workout	**Superset 1**		
			Walking lunge	6–8 or 10–12	Set 1: Set 2:
			Straddle box jump	6–8 or 10–12	Set 1: Set 2:
			Superset 2		
			Straight-leg dead lift	8–10 or 12–15	Set 1: Set 2:
			Switch split jump	6–8 or 10–12	Set 1: Set 2:
			Standing calf raise	10–12 or 15–20	Set 1: Set 2: Set 3:
	Thursday	Rest day			

Friday	Interval CV workout			
	Leg toning workout	**Superset 1**		
		Walking lunge	6–8 or 10–12	Set 1: Set 2:
		Straddle box jump	6–8 or 10–12	Set 1: Set 2:
		Superset 2		
		Straight-leg dead lift	8–10 or 12–15	Set 1: Set 2:
		Switch split jump	6–8 or 10–12	Set 1: Set 2:
		Standing calf raise	10–12 or 15–20	Set 1: Set 2: Set 3:
Saturday	Rest day			
Sunday	Rest day			

5 nutrition

If you want to get leaner legs, you need to eat smart as well as work out regularly. Making a few simple changes to your eating habits will save you calories and help you shed surplus body fat as well as boost your intake of nutrients. And if you have cellulite, this diet plan will help to get rid of the fat deposits that have caused it. If you do not need to lose weight, however, you may require slightly larger portions than are recommended in the five-day plan, or you could supplement this diet with extra snacks that follow the diet guidelines.

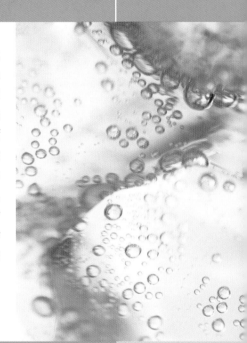

lovely legs nutrition tips

Here are some proven strategies to help you lose those unwanted pounds.

work out before breakfast

If you're working out to lose weight, then exercise before breakfast. This is when your insulin levels are at their lowest, and levels of glucagon – the hormone that helps break down glycogen to energy – are at their highest. And this encourages more fat to leave your fat cells, travel to your muscles and get used for energy.

carb up early

A healthy breakfast kick-starts your metabolism so it works efficiently to burn calories throughout the day. Opt for porridge or high-fibre cereal for a sustained energy boost. Your body is much better at burning carbs in the morning than the evening – one reason why breakfast-eaters maintain a healthy weight more easily than those who skip breakfast.

trim the (bad) fat

It sounds obvious but fat makes you fat. As the fat you eat is close to the form it's stored in if unused, for every 100 calories of fat you eat you use only three to process it. That leaves 97 behind to be burned or stored. Metabolising 100 calories of carbohydrates, on the other hand, requires 10–15 calories, while protein needs 20 calories to make it useable.

eat fish and walnuts

Eat at least one portion of oily fish a week. Try salmon, sardines or mackerel as they're packed with omega-3 fatty acids, which boost your metabolism and promote firm, elastic skin. Alternatively, 25 g (approximately 1 heaped tablespoon) of walnuts or rapeseed oil, or 1–2 omega-3-enriched eggs, will help you meet your daily quota of omega-3 fats.

fruit, not juice

Fruit juice is healthy but actual fruit is better. Down a glass of orange juice and you'll take in about 120 calories, but if you eat an orange instead (60 calories) you'll save calories, get more fibre and still get your daily vitamin C quota.

eat before you shop

Avoid food shopping on an empty stomach or you're more likely to succumb to temptation and fill your trolley with biscuits, cakes and other high-cal goodies. And always make a list before you hit the shops to reduce the risk of making impulse buys.

eat slowly

Sit down and eat slowly rather than on the hoof. People eat up to 15 per cent more calories when they rush at mealtimes. Scoffing your meal means that your hypothalamus – the part of the brain that senses when you are full – doesn't receive the right signals, which explains why you may overeat before feeling full.

fill up on veggies

Eat too many carbs before bedtime and you won't burn all the calories you take in. So pile your plate with vegetables instead of loads of pasta, potatoes and bread. Aim to fill 50 per cent of your plate with veggies (such as carrots, broccoli and salad), 25 per cent with lean protein (such as fish, chicken, dairy or vegetarian protein) and 25 per cent with complex carbohydrates (such as potatoes, rice or pasta).

ditch the fizz

Drinking water rather than sugary fizzy drinks is a great way to cut back on calories, and water won't rot your teeth or leach calcium from your bones. A 500 ml bottle of cola contains 210 calories and 55 g of sugar (equivalent to 11 teaspoons). If you have a daily cola habit it could be costing you 76,650 calories a year – that's enough to put on almost 10 kg (22 lb) of fat!

drink plenty of water

Don't confuse thirst with hunger. Both sensations are remarkably similar so if you don't recognise thirst, you'll assume you're hungry and eat instead of drink. Try drinking a glass of water next time you're peckish and wait 10 minutes. If you feel full, you weren't really hungry, and you won't have taken on board unnecessary calories.

keep it simple

If you're presented with a wide variety of foods you're likely to eat more, according to research from Tuft's University in the US. So when you're faced with a wide array of foods, opt for just two or three types rather than a bit of everything.

bin the crisps

Give up your daily habit of munching a bag of crisps and you'll save 840 calories a week. That's a total of over 3,500 calories saved in a month, or ½ kg (1 lb) of fat lost.

balance your diet

Aim to include the suggested number of portions of each food group every day (see overleaf).

RECOMMENDED DAILY PORTIONS OF EACH FOOD GROUP

Food group	Number of portions each day	Food	Portion size
Vegetables	3–5	**1 portion = 80 g** Broccoli, cauliflower	 2–3 spears/florets
		Carrots	1 carrot
		Peas	3 tablespoons
		Other vegetables	3 tablespoons
		Tomatoes	5 cherry tomatoes
Fruit	2–4	**1 portion = 80 g** Apple, pear, peach, banana	 1 medium fruit
		Plum, kiwi fruit, satsuma	1–2 fruit
		Strawberries	8–10
		Grapes	12–16
		Tinned fruit	3 tablespoons
		Fruit juice	1 medium glass
Grains and potatoes	4–6	Bread	2 slices
		Rolls/muffins	1 roll
		Pasta or rice	6 tablespoons
		Breakfast cereal	1 bowl

		Potatoes, sweet potatoes, yams	Size of your fist
Calcium-rich foods	2–4	Milk (dairy or calcium-fortified soya milk)	1 medium cup
		Cheese	Size of 4 dice
		Tofu	Size of 4 dice
		Tinned sardines	1–2 tablespoons
		Yoghurt/fromage frais	1 pot
Protein-rich foods	2–4	Lean meat	1–2 slices (40–80 g)
		Poultry	2 medium slices/1 breast
		Fish	1 fillet
		Egg	2
		Lentils/beans	Size of your palm
		Tofu/soya burger or sausage	1–2
Healthy fats and oils	1	Nuts and seeds	1 heaped tablespoon
		Seed oils, nut oils	1 tablespoon
		Avocado	Half
		Oily fish*	Deck of cards

*Oily fish is very rich in essential fats so just 1 portion a week would cover your needs

five-day eating plan

Use this five-day plan as the basis for developing your own eating plan. Each day, aim to have three meals with two healthy snacks in between. And don't forget to drink at least six to eight glasses of water or fruit/herbal tea a day.

fruit portions

Where one portion of fruit is indicated on the menu, select one from this list. Vary your choices so you get more nutrients.

1 medium fruit: apples, oranges, bananas, peaches, pears

2 small fruit: satsumas, apricots, plums, kiwi fruit

1 cupful (125 g) of berry-type fruit: grapes, strawberries, raspberries, cherries

½ large fruit: mangos, papayas, grapefruits

1 glass fruit juice: all 100 per cent fruit juices (not fruit drinks)

day 1 menu plan

breakfast

Porridge made with skimmed milk
1 tablespoon (15 ml) raisins and 3–4 chopped apricots

lunch

Carrot Soup with Fresh Coriander
1 wholemeal roll
1 portion of fresh fruit

evening meal

Pan-fried Salmon with Rocket and Tomato
175 g steamed green vegetables (e.g. broccoli or Brussels sprouts)

snacks

rice crackers (rice cakes) topped with 2 teaspoons (10 ml)
peanut butter
portion fresh fruit

carrot soup with fresh coriander
(makes 1 serving)

■ Heat 1 tablespoon (15 ml) extra virgin olive oil in a heavy-based saucepan over a moderate heat. Add half an onion, finely sliced, and sauté gently for about 5 minutes until translucent.

■ Add half a crushed garlic clove and cook for a further 1–2 minutes. Then add 2 sliced carrots, 250 ml vegetable stock and a bay leaf to the pan, stir, and bring to the boil. Simmer for 15 minutes or until the vegetables are tender.

■ Allow the soup to cool slightly for a couple of minutes. Remove and discard the bay leaf. Liquidise the soup using a hand blender or conventional blender. Season to taste with low-sodium salt and pepper, then stir in a handful of roughly chopped fresh coriander.

pan-fried salmon with rocket and tomato
(makes 1 serving)

■ Brush a salmon fillet (about 175 g) with a little olive oil. Heat a non-stick pan until hot. Add the salmon and fry for 4–5 minutes, then turn it over and cook the other side for 3 minutes. Remove from the heat.

■ Toss 60 g of vine-ripened baby tomatoes in 1 tablespoon (15 ml) olive oil vinaigrette (homemade or bought). Add a handful of rocket, mix and pile on to a serving plate. Place the salmon on top and serve immediately.

Vegetarian: Substitute a nut burger or cutlet and 25 g walnuts for the salmon. Cook the nut burger according to the packet instructions. Place on top of the tomato and rocket salad and scatter over 25 g walnuts.

day 2 menu plan

breakfast

Mix 125 g fresh fruit (e.g. chopped mango, sliced bananas, strawberries, raspberries or blueberries) with 150 ml natural bio yoghurt and 1–2 level teaspoons (5–10 ml) honey

lunch

1 small baked potato with a drizzle of extra virgin olive oil
1 tablespoon (15 ml) hummus
Bowl of salad leaves with a drizzle of olive oil dressing
A few walnuts or flaked almonds
1 portion of fresh fruit

evening meal

Pasta with Stir-fried Chicken (or Tofu) and Spring Vegetables
1 portion of fresh fruit.

snacks

60 g dried fruit (e.g. apricots, prunes, peaches, mango)
Small handful of cashews, peanuts or walnuts

pasta with stir-fried chicken (or tofu) and spring vegetables
(makes 2 servings)

▧ Heat 1 tablespoon (15 ml) extra virgin olive oil in a pan and cook 1 clove of crushed garlic and 1 small chopped onion for 3 minutes until softened. Add 85 g cooked, skinless chicken pieces or tofu and continue cooking for 5 minutes.

▧ Steam or boil in a minimal quantity of water 85 g trimmed mangetout, 85 g broccoli florets and 85 g baby spinach leaves for 3–4 minutes until tender-crisp. Drain immediately.

▧ Meanwhile, cook 175 g whole-wheat pasta shapes in boiling water according to the packet instructions. Drain, then combine with the cooked vegetables and chicken (or tofu) mixture. Add a small handful of fresh, chopped mint leaves, season with low-sodium salt and pepper, toss well and serve immediately.

day 3 menu plan

breakfast

50 g muesli with fruit and nuts
125 ml skimmed milk or plain yoghurt

lunch

Broccoli and Courgette Soup with Toasted Almonds
Slice of wholewheat bread
1 portion of fresh fruit

evening meal

Roasted Root Vegetables with Thyme
100 g poached salmon OR 60 g toasted pine nuts or walnuts

Fresh fruit salad with 2 tablespoons plain yoghurt

snacks

125 g fresh fruit (e.g. satsumas or clementines)
Small handful of toasted seeds (e.g. pumpkin, sunflower or sesame seeds)

broccoli and courgette soup with toasted almonds
(makes 2 servings)

- Cook a small, finely chopped onion gently in 1 tablespoon (15 ml) extra virgin olive oil for 5 minutes. Then add 125 g broccoli, divided into small florets, and 225 g sliced courgettes, cover and cook for a further 4–5 minutes until the vegetables are tender.

- Blend 1 tablespoon (15 ml) cornflour with a little water and add to the vegetables, stirring continuously. When blended, add 500 ml vegetable stock. Bring to the boil, stirring, and simmer gently for 1–2 minutes.

- Put the soup into a blender with a little low-sodium salt, freshly ground black pepper and nutmeg and whiz until smooth. Toast 25 g flaked almonds under the grill. Ladle the soup into bowls, and sprinkle with the almonds.

roasted root vegetables with thyme
(makes 2 servings)

▨ Preheat the oven to 200°C/400°F/Gas Mark 6. Prepare the vegetables: peel 1 small sweet potato and cut into wedges; peel 1 parsnip and cut into quarters; peel ¼ swede and cut into wedges; peel ½ small butternut squash and slice thickly. Place in a large roasting tin.

▨ Scatter over a crushed clove of garlic, a few sprigs of fresh thyme, a little low-sodium salt and freshly ground black pepper. Drizzle over 1–2 tablespoons (15–30 ml) olive oil and turn the vegetables gently to coat them.

▨ Roast in the oven for 30–40 minutes until the vegetables are tender.

day 4 menu plan

breakfast

45 g bran flakes (or other bran/wholegrain cereal) topped with a sliced banana and served with 125 ml skimmed or semi-skimmed milk

lunch

Half an avocado
Mixed salad of salad leaves, tomato, yellow pepper and radish
85 g cooked peeled prawns OR 2 tablespoons (30 ml) hummus

evening meal

Stir-fried Vegetables with Turkey (or Tofu) and Cashews
2 heaped tablespoons (30 ml) cooked brown rice

snacks

1 pot natural bio yoghurt mixed with 3 chopped dried apricots
1 portion fresh fruit

stir-fried vegetables with turkey (or tofu) and cashews
(makes 2 servings)

■ Heat 1 tablespoon (15 ml) olive oil in a non-stick wok or large frying pan. Add 125 g turkey breast, cut into strips OR tofu cut into 1-cm cubes and stir-fry for 3–4 minutes. Remove from the pan. Add 1 small sliced onion, 1 teaspoon (5 ml) grated fresh ginger and 1 crushed garlic clove and stir-fry for 2 minutes.

■ Add 85 g broccoli florets, 85 g trimmed thin green beans and 1 sliced courgette and stir-fry for a further 2–3 minutes.

■ Add 125 g bean sprouts, 1 tablespoon (15 ml) water, 1 tablespoon (15 ml) light soy sauce and continue stir-frying for a further minute. Stir in the turkey or tofu and 60g toasted cashew nuts and serve.

day 5 menu plan

breakfast

Slice of wholewheat bread or toast with a little olive oil spread and honey
1 portion of fresh fruit

lunch

Salad leaves with fresh herbs and a few walnuts
150 g steamed or grilled cod steak OR 60 g hummus
125 g fresh fruit

evening meal

Spiced Lentils with Vegetables and Coriander
2 heaped tablespoons (30 ml) cooked brown rice
225 g steamed vegetables (e.g. carrots, broccoli, courgettes, green beans)

snacks

1 pot (150 g) plain yoghurt with a little honey (optional)
2 rye crackers with 2 tablespoons (30ml) cottage cheese

spiced lentils with vegetables and coriander
(makes 2 servings)

■ Heat 1–2 tablespoons (15–30 ml) olive oil in a heavy-based pan and sauté a chopped onion for 5 minutes. Add a crushed clove of garlic, $\frac{1}{2}$ teaspoon (2.5 ml) ground cumin and 1 teaspoon (5 ml) ground coriander, and continue cooking for 1 minute.

■ Add 85 g red lentils, 400 ml vegetable stock and 2 diced small carrots. Bring to the boil. Cover and simmer for about 20 minutes, adding 125 g frozen peas 5 minutes before the end of the cooking time.

■ Stir in 1 tablespoon (15 ml) lemon juice and a little low-sodium salt. Finally, stir in a small handful of freshly chopped coriander.

6 maintenance

Congratulations on reaching the end of this six-week programme. Hopefully, you have now achieved your initial goals and are pleased with your results.

moving on

This six-week programme has introduced you to new exercises, and helped you to establish new diet and activity habits. But the programme doesn't end just because the book does. Give yourself a short break from the plan – I suggest a week – then decide on your next goal. You can either repeat this programme or incorporate any of the exercises into a longer-term workout and diet plan to maintain your lovely legs and your overall fitness.

Stick to the following principles:

- Aim to complete three CV workouts for a minimum of 20 minutes each week.

- Vary your activity as often as possible to increase your calorie burn, boost your motivation and reduce injury risk.

- Monitor your heart rate or use your RPE to ensure you are continually challenging your body – make sure that you push yourself hard enough every workout.

- Aim to complete a leg-toning workout twice a week. Choose any of the six workouts in this book and try to vary the exercises you do as much as possible.

- Try to leave at least one day between workouts.

- Reread 'Exercise Tips' on pages 3–5 to make sure you don't lapse into bad habits.

- Continue to eat smart – reread the tips in Chapter 5 and use the diet plans and meal suggestions for the basis of your eating plan.

Best wishes and good luck!

index